The Vibrant Cooking Guide to Keto Pasta

A Collection of Super Easy and Affordable Low Carb Recipes to Boost Your Metabolism

Skye Webb

Table of contents

Zucchini Vegan Bacon Lasagna

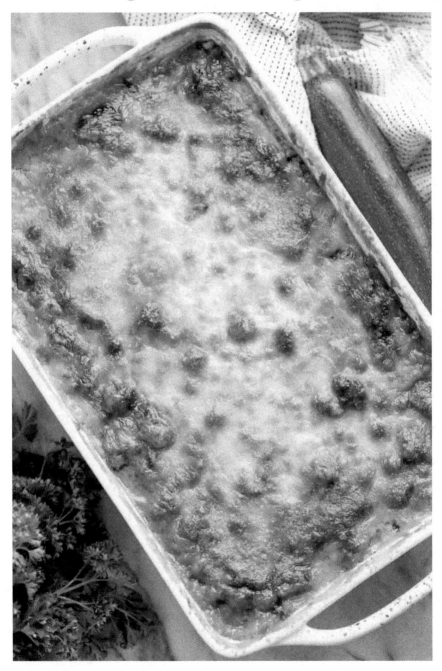

Preparation Time: 15 minutes Cooking Time: 40 minutes Serving: 4

Ingredients:

4 large yellow zucchinis

Salt and black pepper to taste

1 tbsp lard

½ lb vegan bacon 1 tsp garlic powder

1 tsp onion powder

2 tbsp coconut flour

1   ½ cup grated mozzarella cheese

1/3 cup cheddar cheese

2   cups crumbled ricotta cheese

1 large egg

2 cups unsweetened marinara sauce

1 tbsp Italian herb seasoning

¼ tsp red chili flakes

¼ cup fresh basil leaves

Directions:

1.   Preheat the oven to 375 F and grease a 9 x 9-inch baking dish with cooking spray. Set aside.

2.   Slice the zucchini into ¼ -inch strips, arrange on a flat surface and sprinkle generously with salt. Set aside to release

liquid for 5 to 10 minutes. Pat dry with a paper towel and set aside.

3.   Melt the lard in a large skillet over medium heat and add the vegan bacon. Cook until browned, 10 minutes. Set aside to cool.

4.   In a medium bowl, evenly combine the garlic powder, onion powder, coconut flour, salt, black pepper, mozzarella cheese, half of the cheddar cheese, ricotta cheese, and egg. Set aside.

5.   Add the Italian herb seasoning and red chili flakes to the marinara sauce and mix. Set aside.

6.   Make a single layer of the zucchini in the baking dish; spread a quarter of the egg mixture on top, and a quarter of the marinara sauce. Repeat the layering process and sprinkle the top with the remaining cheddar cheese.

7.   Bake in the oven for 30 minutes or until golden brown on top.

8.   Remove the dish from the oven, allow cooling for 5 to 10 minutes, garnish with the basil leaves, slice and serve.

Nutrition: Calories:417, Total Fat: 36.4g, Saturated Fat: 15.9g, Total Carbs: 4g, Dietary Fiber:0g, Sugar: 1g, Protein20: g, Sodium: 525mg

Parsley-Lime Pasta

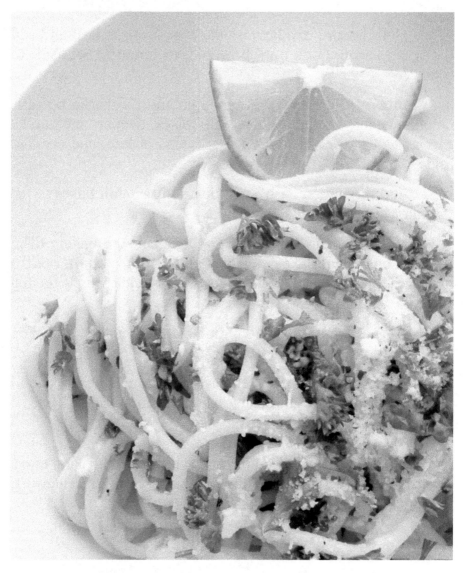

Preparation Time: 20 minutes Serving: 4

Ingredients:

2 tbsp butter

1 lb tempeh, chopped

4 garlic cloves, minced

1 pinch red chili flakes

¼ cup white wine

1 lime, zested and juiced

3 medium zucchinis, spiralized

 Salt and black pepper to taste

2 tbsp chopped parsley

1 cup grated parmesan cheese for topping

Directions:

1.   Melt the butter in a large skillet and cook in the tempeh until golden brown.

2.   Flip and stir in the garlic and red chili flakes. Cook further for 1 minute; transfer to a plate and set aside.

3.   Pour the wine and lime juice into the skillet, and cook until reduced by a quarter. Meanwhile, stir to deglaze the bottom of the pot.

4.   Mix in the zucchinis, lime zest, tempeh and parsley. Season with salt and black pepper, and toss everything well. Cook until the zucchinis is slightly tender for 2 minutes.

5.   Dish the food onto serving plates and top generously with the parmesan cheese.

Nutrition: Calories: 326, Total Fat: 24.9g, Saturated Fat:12.9 g, Total Carbs: 6 g, Dietary Fiber:1g, Sugar: 4g, Protein: 20g, Sodium: 568mg

Creamy Garlic Mushrooms with Angel Hair Shirataki

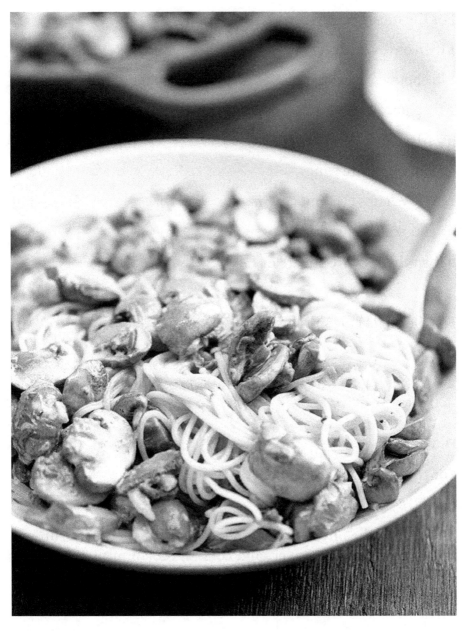

Preparation Time: 25 minutes Serving: 4

Ingredients:

For the mushroom sauce:

1 tbsp olive oil

1 lb chopped mushrooms Salt and black pepper to taste

2 tbsp unsalted butter

6 garlic cloves, minced

½ cup dry white wine

1   ½ cups coconut cream

½ cup grated parmesan cheese

2 tbsp chopped fresh parsley

For the angel hair shirataki:

2   (8 oz) packs angel hair shirataki noodles Salt to season

Directions:

For the mushroom sauce:

1.   Heat the olive oil in a large skillet, season the mushroom with salt and black pepper, and cook in the oil until softened, 5 minutes. Transfer to a plate and set aside.

2.   Melt the butter in the skillet and sauté the garlic until fragrant. Stir in the white wine and cook until reduced by half, meanwhile, scraping the bottom of the pan to deglaze.

3.   Reduce the heat to low and stir in the coconut cream. Allow simmering for 1 minute and stir in the parmesan cheese to melt.

4.   Return the mushroom to the sauce and sprinkle the parsley on top. Adjust the taste with salt and black pepper, if needed.

For the angel hair shirataki:

5.   Bring 2 cups of water to a boil in a medium pot over medium heat.

6.   Strain the shirataki pasta through a colander and rinse very well under hot running water.

7.   Allow proper draining and pour the shirataki pasta into the boiling water. Cook for 3 minutes and strain again.

8.   Place a dry skillet over medium heat and stir-fry the shirataki pasta until visibly dry and makes a squeaky sound when stirred, 1 to 2 minutes.

9.   Season with salt and plate.

10.   Top the shirataki pasta with the mushroom sauce and serve warm.

Nutrition: Calories:89, Total Fat:6.4 g, Saturated Fat:1.5 g, Total Carbs: 2g, Dietary Fiber:0g, Sugar:1g, Protein:6 g, Sodium: 406mg

Coconut Tofu Zucchini Bake

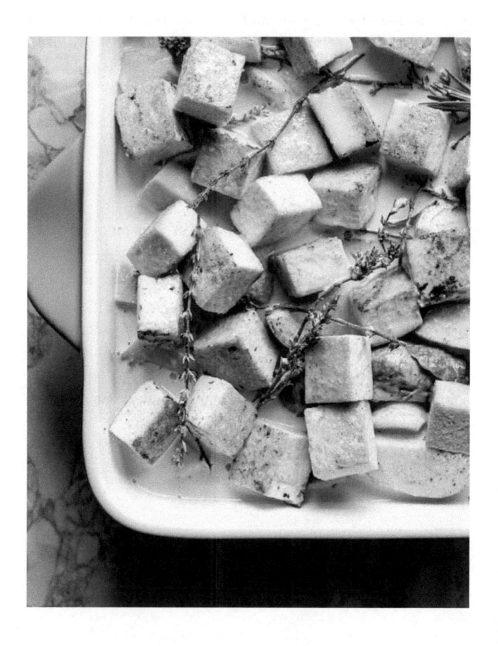

Preparation Time: 40 minutes Serving: 4

Ingredients:

1 tbsp butter

1 cup green beans, chopped

1   bunch asparagus, trimmed and cut into 1-inch pieces

2 tbsp arrowroot starch

2   cups coconut milk

4 medium zucchinis, spiralized

1 cup grated parmesan cheese

1   (15 oz) firm tofu, pressed and sliced

Salt and black pepper to taste

Directions:

1.   Preheat the oven to 380 F.

2.   Melt the butter in a medium skillet and sauté the green beans and asparagus until softened, about 5 minutes. Set aside.

3.   In a medium saucepan, mix the arrowroot starch with the coconut milk. Bring to a boil over medium heat with frequent stirring until thickened, 3 minutes. Stir in half of the parmesan cheese until melted.

4.   Mix in the green beans, asparagus, zucchinis and tofu. Season with salt and black pepper.

5.   Transfer the mixture to a baking dish and cover the top with the remaining parmesan cheese.

6.   Bake in the oven until the cheese melts and golden on top, 20 minutes.

7.   Remove the food from the oven and serve warm.

Nutrition: Calories: 492, Total Fat:26.8 g, Saturated Fat: 12.6g, Total Carbs: 14g, Dietary Fiber:4g, Sugar: 8g, Protein: 50g, Sodium: 1668mg

Creamy Seitan Shirataki Fettucine

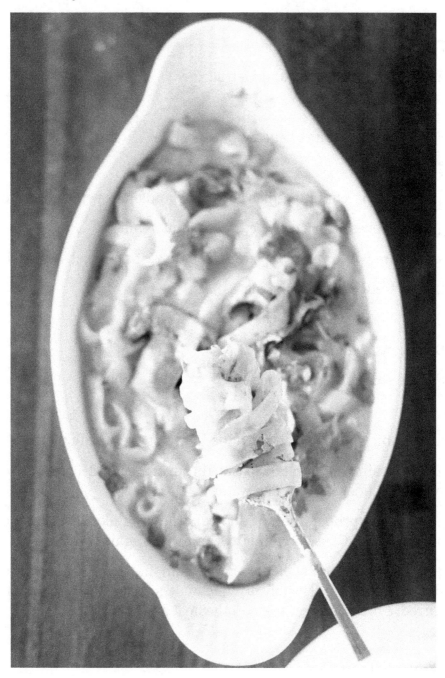

Preparation Time: 35 minutes Serving: 4

Ingredients:

For the shirataki fettuccine:

2   (8 oz) packs shirataki fettuccine

For the creamy seitan sauce:

5 tbsp butter

4 seitan slabs, cut into 2-inch cubes Salt and black pepper to taste

3 garlic cloves, minced 1 ¼ cups coconut cream

½ cup dry white wine 1 tsp grated lemon zest 1 cup baby spinach

Lemon wedges for garnishing

Directions:

For the shirataki fettuccine:

1.   Boil 2 cups of water in a medium pot over medium heat.

2.   Strain the shirataki pasta through a colander and rinse very well under hot running water.

3.   Allow proper draining and pour the shirataki pasta into the boiling water. Cook for 3 minutes and strain again.

4.   Place a dry skillet over medium heat and stir-fry the shirataki pasta until visibly dry, and makes a squeaky sound when stirred, 1 to 2 minutes. Take off the heat and set aside.

For the seitan sauce:

5.   Melt half of the butter in a large skillet; season the seitan with salt, black pepper, and cook in the butter until golden brown on all sides and flaky within, 8 minutes. Transfer to a plate and set aside.

6.   Add the remaining butter to the skillet to melt and stir in the garlic. Cook until fragrant, 1 minute.

7.   Mix in the coconut cream, white wine, lemon zest, salt, and black pepper. Allow boiling over low heat until the sauce thickens, 5 minutes.

8.   Stir in the spinach, allow wilting for 2 minutes and stir in the shirataki fettuccine and seitan until well- coated in the sauce. Adjust the taste with salt and black pepper.

9.   Dish the food and garnish with the lemon wedges. Serve warm.

Nutrition: Calories: 720, Total Fat: 56.5g, Saturated Fat: 27.2g, Total Carbs: 17 g, Dietary Fiber:3g, Sugar: 7g, Protein: 37g, Sodium:1764 mg

Tofu and Spinach Lasagna with Red Sauce

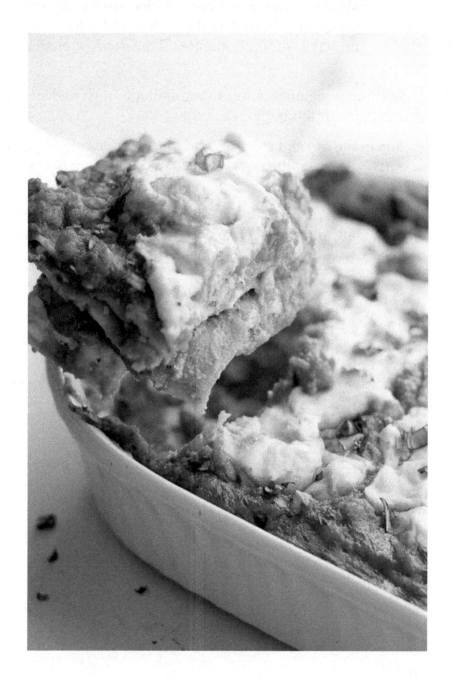

Preparation Time: 20minutes Cooking Time: 45minutes Serving: 4

Ingredients:

2 tbsp butter

1 white onion, chopped

1 garlic clove, minced

2 ½ cups crumbled tofu

3 tbsp tomato paste

½ tbsp dried oregano

1 tsp salt

¼ tsp ground black pepper

½ cup water

1 cup baby spinach

For the low-carb pasta:

Flax egg: 8 tbsp flax seed powder + 1 ½ cups water

1 ½ cup dairy-free cashew cream

1 tsp salt

5 tbsp psyllium husk powder

For topping:

2 cups coconut cream

5 oz. shredded mozzarella cheese

2 oz. grated tofu cheese

½ tsp salt

¼ tsp ground black pepper

½ cup fresh parsley, finely chopped

Directions:

1.	Melt the butter in a medium pot over medium heat. Then, add the white onion and garlic, and sauté until fragrant and soft, about 3 minutes.

2.	Stir in the tofu and cook until brown. Mix in the tomato paste, oregano, salt, and black pepper.

3.	Pour the water into the pot, stir, and simmer the Ingredients until most of the liquid has evaporated.

4.	While cooking the sauce, make the lasagna sheets. Preheat the oven to 300 F and mix the flax seed powder with the water in a medium bowl to make flax egg. Allow sitting to thicken for 5 minutes.

5.	Combine the flax egg with the cashew cream and salt. Add the psyllium husk powder a bit at a time while whisking and allow the mixture to sit for a few more minutes.

6.	Line a baking sheet with parchment paper and spread the mixture in. Cover with another parchment paper and use a rolling pin to flatten the dough into the sheet.

7.	Bake the batter in the oven for 10 to 12 minutes, remove after, take off the parchment papers, and slice the pasta into sheets that fit your baking dish.

8.   In a bowl, combine the coconut cream and two-thirds of the mozzarella cheese. Fetch out 2 tablespoons of the mixture and reserve.

9.   Mix in the tofu cheese, salt, black pepper, and parsley. Set aside.

10.   Grease your baking dish with cooking spray and lay in one-third of the pasta sheet; spread half of the tomato sauce on top, add another one-third set of the pasta sheets, the remaining tomato sauce and the rest of the pasta sheets.

11.   Grease your baking dish with cooking spray, layer a single line of pasta in the dish, spread with some tomato sauce, 1/3 of the spinach, and ¼ of the coconut cream mixture. Season with salt and black pepper as desired.

12.   Repeat layering the Ingredients twice in the same manner making sure to top the final layer with the coconut cream mixture and the reserved cashew cream.

13.   Bake in the oven for 30 minutes at 400 F or until the lasagna has a beautiful

brown surface.

14.   Remove the dish; allow cooling for a few minutes, and slice.

15.   Serve the lasagna with a baby green salad.

Nutrition: Calories: 487, Total Fat:45.3g, Saturated Fat:34.2g, Total Carbs: 13g, Dietary Fiber:3g, Sugar: 2g, Protein: 14g, Sodium:459 mg

Zoodle Bolognese

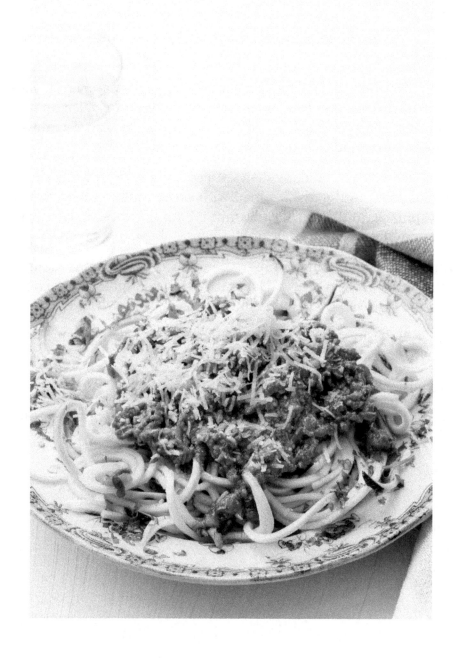

Preparation Time: 10minutes Cooking Time: 35minutes Serving: 4

Ingredients:

For the Bolognese sauce:

3 oz. olive oil

1 white onion, chopped

1 garlic clove, minced

3 oz. celery, chopped

3 cups crumbled tofu

2 tbsp tomato paste

1 ½ cups crushed tomatoes

1 tsp salt

¼ tsp black pepper

1 tbsp dried basil

1 tbsp Worcestershire sauce

Water as needed

For the zoodles:

1   lb zucchinis

2   tbsp butter

Salt and black pepper to taste

Directions:

1.   Pour the olive oil into a saucepan and heat over medium heat. When no longer shimmering, add the onion, garlic, and celery. Sauté for 3 minutes or until the onions are soft and the carrots caramelized.

2.   Pour in the tofu, tomato paste, tomatoes, salt, black pepper, basil, and Worcestershire sauce. Stir and cook for 15 minutes, or simmer for 30 minutes.

3.   Mix in some water if the mixture is too thick and simmer further for 20 minutes.

4.   While the sauce cooks, make the zoodles. Run the zucchini through a spiralizer to form noodles.

5.   Melt the butter in a skillet over medium heat and toss the zoodles quickly in the butter, about 1 minute only.

6.   Season with salt and black pepper.

Nutrition: Calories: ,239 Total Fat:14.7g, Saturated Fat:8.1g, Total Carbs: 14g, Dietary Fiber:1g, Sugar:7 g, Protein: 13g, Sodium: 530mg

Creamy Mushrooms with Shirataki

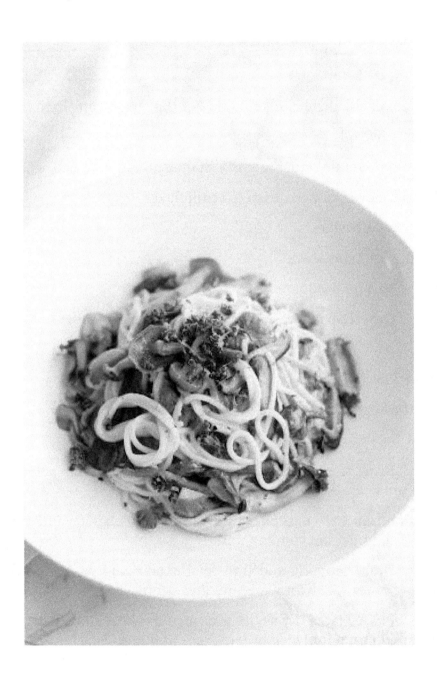

Preparation Time: 25 minutes Serving: 4

Ingredients:

For the angel hair shirataki:

2 (8 oz) packs angel hair shirataki For the creamy mushrooms:

4 tbsp olive oil

1 lb sliced cremini mushrooms 3 shallots, finely chopped

6 garlic cloves, minced 2 tsp red chili flakes

¼ cup white wine

½ cup vegetable stock

1   ½ cups coconut cream

2   tbsp chopped fresh parsley Salt and black pepper to taste

Directions:

For the angel hair shirataki:

1.   Bring 2 cups of water to a boil in a medium pot over medium heat.

2.   Strain the shirataki pasta through a colander and rinse very well under hot running water.

3.   Drain properly and transfer the shirataki pasta into the boiling water. Cook for 3 minutes and strain again.

4.   Place a large dry skillet over medium heat and stir-fry the shirataki pasta until visibly dry, 1 to 2 minutes. Take off the heat and set aside.

For the creamy mushrooms:

5.   Heat the olive oil in a large skillet and sauté the mushrooms, shallots, garlic, and chili flakes until softened and fragrant, 3 minutes.

6.   Mix in the white wine and vegetable stock. Allow boiling and whisk in the remaining butter and then the coconut cream.

7.   Taste the sauce and adjust the taste with salt, black pepper, and mix in the parsley.

8.   Pour in the shirataki pasta, mussels and toss well in the sauce.

9.   Serve afterwards.

Nutrition: Calories:673, Total Fat:58.8g, Saturated Fat:36.3g, Total Carbs: 16g, Dietary Fiber:7, Sugar:2 g, Protein: 26g, Sodium:760 mg

Tempeh Alfredo Squash Spaghetti

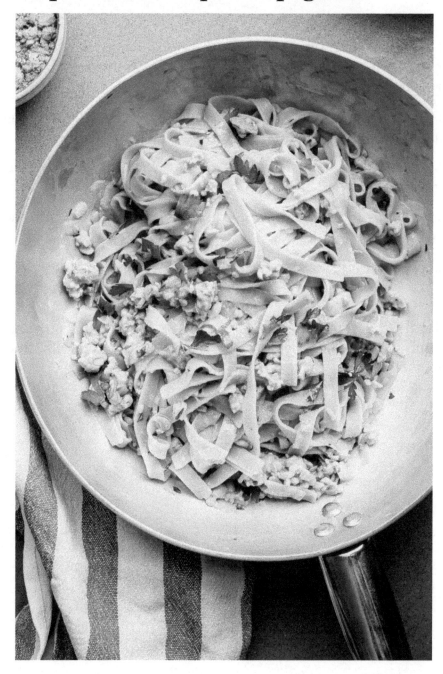

Preparation Time: 1 hour and 20 minutes Serving: 4

Ingredients:

For the pasta:

2 medium spaghetti squashes, halved 2 tbsp olive oil

For the sauce:

2 tbsp butter

1 lb tempeh, crumbled

½ tsp garlic powder

Salt and black pepper to taste 1 tsp arrowroot starch

1 ½ cups coconut cream A pinch of nutmeg

1/3 cup finely grated parmesan cheese

1/3 cup finely grated tempeh mozzarella cheese

Directions:

1.   Preheat the oven to 375 F and line a baking dish with foil. Set aside.

2.   Season the squash with the olive oil, salt, and black pepper. Place the squash on the baking dish, open side up and roast for 45 to 50 minutes until the squash is tender.

3. When ready, remove the squash from the oven, allow cooling and use two forks to shred the inner part of the noodles. Set aside.

4. Melt the butter in a medium pot, add the tempeh, garlic powder, salt, and black pepper, cook until brown, 10 minutes.

5. Stir in the arrowroot starch, coconut cream, and nutmeg. Cook until the sauce thickens, 2 to 3 minutes.

6. Spoon the sauce into the squashes and cover with the parmesan and mozzarella cheeses.

7. Place under the oven's broiler and cook until the cheeses melt and golden brown, 2 to 3 minutes.

8. Remove from the oven and serve warm.

Nutrition: Calories:865, Total Fat:80.2g, Saturated Fat:56.8g, Total Carbs: 19g, Dietary Fiber:5g, Sugar: 5g, Protein: 28g, Sodium: 1775mg

Keto Pasta with Mediterranean Tofu balls

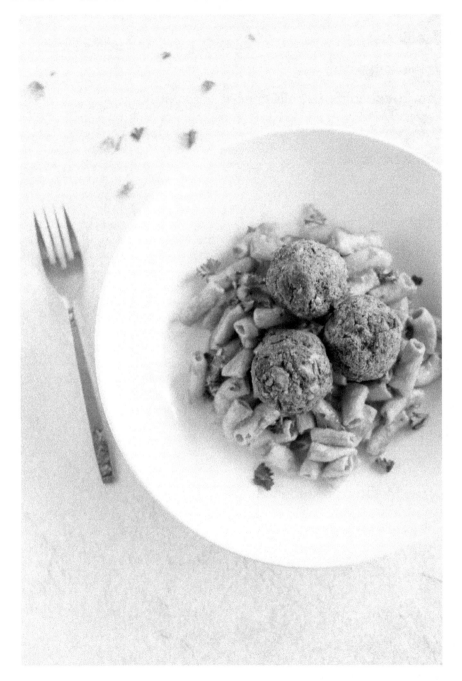

Preparation Time: 90 minutes + overnight chilling Serving size: 4

Ingredients:

For the keto pasta:

1 cup shredded mozzarella cheese 1 egg yolk

For the sauce:

3 tbsp olive oil

2 yellow onions, chopped

6 garlic cloves, minced

2 tbsp unsweetened tomato paste

2 large tomatoes, chopped

¼ tsp saffron powder

2 cinnamon sticks

4 ½ cups vegetable broth

Salt and black pepper to taste

For the Mediterranean meatballs:

2 cups mushroom rinds 1 lb tofu

1 egg

¼ cup almond milk

6 garlic cloves, minced

Salt and black pepper to taste

½ tsp coriander powder

¼ tsp nutmeg powder 1 tbsp smoked paprika

1 ½ tsp fresh ginger paste 1 tsp cumin powder

½ tsp cayenne pepper

1 ½ tsp turmeric powder

½ tsp cloves powder

4 tbsp chopped cilantro 4 tbsp chopped scallions 4 tbsp chopped parsley

¼ cup almond flour

¼ cup olive oil

1   cup crumbled cottage cheese for serving

Directions:

For the pasta:

1.   Pour the cheese into a medium safe-microwave bowl and melt in the microwave for 35 minutes or until melted.

2.   Remove the bowl and allow cooling for 1 minute only to warm the cheese but not cool completely. Mix in the egg yolk until well combined.

3.   Lay parchment paper on a flat surface, pour the cheese mixture on top and cover with another parchment paper. Using a rolling pin, flatten the dough into 1/8-inch thickness.

4.   Take off the parchment paper and cut the dough into spaghetti strands. Place in a bowl and refrigerate overnight.

5.   When ready to cook, bring 2 cups of water to a boil in a medium saucepan and add the pasta.

6.   Cook for 40 seconds to 1 minute and then drain through a colander. Run cold water over the pasta and set aside to cool.

For the Mediterranean tofu balls:

7.   In a large pot, heat the olive oil and sauté the onions until softened, 3 minutes. Stir in the garlic and cook until fragrant, 30 seconds.

8.   Stir in the tomato paste, tomatoes, saffron, and cinnamon sticks; cook for 2 minutes and then mix in the vegetable broth, salt, and black pepper. Simmer for 20 to 25 minutes while you make the tofu balls.

9.   In a large bowl, mix the mushroom rinds, tofu, egg, almond milk, garlic, salt, black pepper, coriander, nutmeg powder, paprika, ginger paste, cumin powder, cayenne pepper, turmeric powder, cloves powder, cilantro, parsley, 3 tablespoons of scallions, and almond flour. Form 1-inch meatballs from the mixture.

10.   Heat the olive oil in a large skillet and fry the tofu balls in batches until brown on all sides, 10 minutes.

11.   Put the tofu balls into the sauce, coat well with the sauce and continue cooking over low heat for 5 to 10 minutes.

12.   Divide the pasta onto serving plates and spoon the tofu balls with sauce on top.

13.   Garnish with the cottage cheese, remaining scallions and serve warm.

Nutrition: Calories: 232, Total Fat:14.3g, Saturated Fat:5.4g, Total Carbs: 12g, Dietary Fiber:g4, Sugar:4 g, Protein:20 g, Sodium: 719mg

Seitan-Asparagus Shirataki Mix

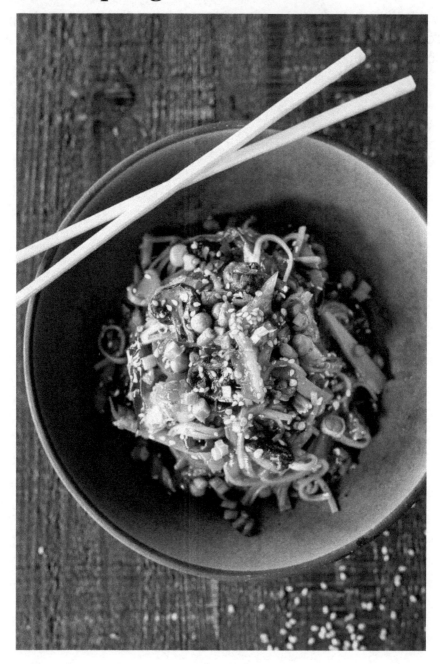

Preparation Time: 40 minutes Serving: 4

Ingredients:

For the angel hair shirataki:

2   (8 oz) packs angel hair shirataki

For the seitan-asparagus base:

1 lb seitan

3 tbsp olive oil

1 lb fresh asparagus, cut into 1-inch pieces 2 large shallots, finely chopped

3 garlic cloves, minced

Salt and black pepper to taste

1   cup finely grated parmesan cheese for topping

Directions:

For the angel hair shirataki:

1.   Bring 2 cups of water to a boil in a medium pot over medium heat.

2.   Strain the shirataki pasta through a colander and rinse very well under hot running water.

3.   Drain properly and transfer the shirataki pasta into the boiling water. Cook for 3 minutes and strain again.

4.   Place a dry large skillet over medium heat and stir-fry the shirataki pasta until visibly dry, 1 to 2 minutes. Take off the heat and set aside.

For the seitan -asparagus base:

5.   Heat a large non-stick skillet over medium heat and add the seitan. Cook while breaking the lumps that form until brown, 10 minutes. Use a slotted spoon to transfer the seitan to a plate and discard the drippings.

6.   Heat the olive oil in the skillet and sauté the asparagus until tender, 5 to 7 minutes. Stir in the shallots and garlic and cook until fragrant, 2 minutes. Season with salt and black pepper.

7.   Stir in the seitan, shirataki and toss until well combined. Adjust the taste with salt and black pepper as desired.

8.   Dish the food onto serving plates and garnish generously with the parmesan cheese.

9.   Serve warm.

Nutrition: Calories:413, Total Fat:30.6g, Saturated Fat:12.3g, Total Carbs: 8g, Dietary Fiber:2g, Sugar: 4g, Protein:5 g, Sodium:37 mg

Garlic-Butter Tempeh with Shirataki Fettucine

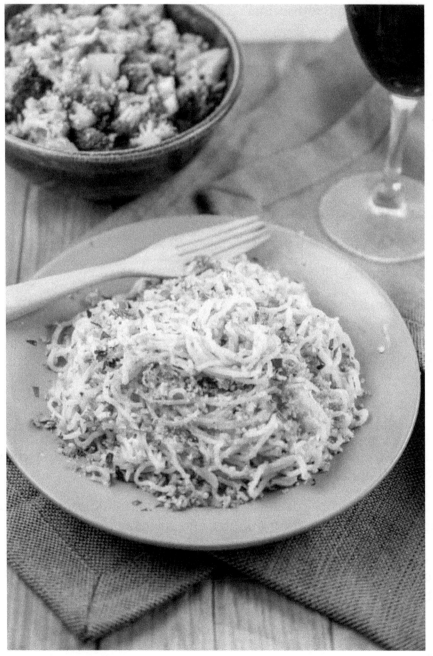

Preparation Time: 30 minutes Serving: 4

Ingredients:

For the shirataki fettuccine:

2   (8 oz) packs shirataki fettuccine For the garlic-butter steak bites:

4 tbsp butter

1 lb thick-cut tempeh, cut into 1-inch cubes

Salt and black pepper to taste

4 garlic cloves, mined

2 tbsp chopped fresh parsley

1   cup freshly grated parmesan cheese

Directions:

For the shirataki fettuccine:

1.   Boil 2 cups of water in a medium pot over medium heat.

2.   Strain the shirataki pasta through a colander and rinse very well under hot running water.

3.   Allow proper draining and pour the shirataki pasta into the boiling water. Cook for 3 minutes and strain again.

4.   Place a dry skillet over medium heat and stir-fry the shirataki pasta until visibly dry, and makes a squeaky sound when stirred, 1 to 2 minutes. Take off the heat and set aside.

For the garlic-butter mushroom bites:

5.   Melt the butter in a large skillet, season the mushroom with salt, black pepper and cook in the butter until brown, and cooked through, 10 minutes.

6.   Stir in the garlic and cook until fragrant, 1 minute.

7.   Mix in the parsley and shirataki pasta; toss well and season with salt and black pepper.

8.   Dish the food, top with the parmesan cheese and serve immediately.

Nutrition: Calories:399, Total Fat: 34.2g, Saturated Fat: 18.6g, Total Carbs: 10 g, Dietary Fiber:0g, Sugar: 2g, Protein:17 g, Sodium: 283mg

Eggplant Ragu

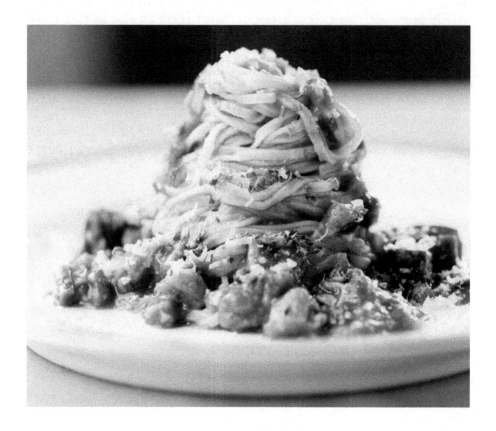

Preparation Time: 20 minutes Serving: 4

Ingredients

2   tbsp butter

1 lb eggplant

Salt and black pepper to taste

1 / 4 cup sugar-free tomato sauce

4 tbsp chopped fresh parsley + extra for garnishing

4 large green bell peppers, Blade A, noodles trimmed

4 large red bell peppers, Blade A, noodles trimmed

1 small red onion, Blade A, noodles trimmed

1 cup grated parmesan cheese

Directions:

1.   Heat half of the butter in a medium skillet and cook the eggplant until brown, 5 minutes. Season with salt and black pepper.

2.   Stir in the tomato sauce, parsley, and cook for 10 minutes or until the sauce reduces by a quarter.

3.   Stir in the bell pepper and onion noodles; cook for 1 minute and turn the heat off.

4.   Adjust the taste with salt, black pepper, and dish the food onto serving plates.

5.   Garnish with the parmesan cheese and more parsley; serve warm.

Nutrition: Calories: 163, Total Fat: 9.8g, Saturated Fat:5.6 g, Total Carbs: 7 g, Dietary Fiber:2g, Sugar:4g, Protein: 13g, Sodium: 417mg

Thai Tofu Shirataki Stir-Fry

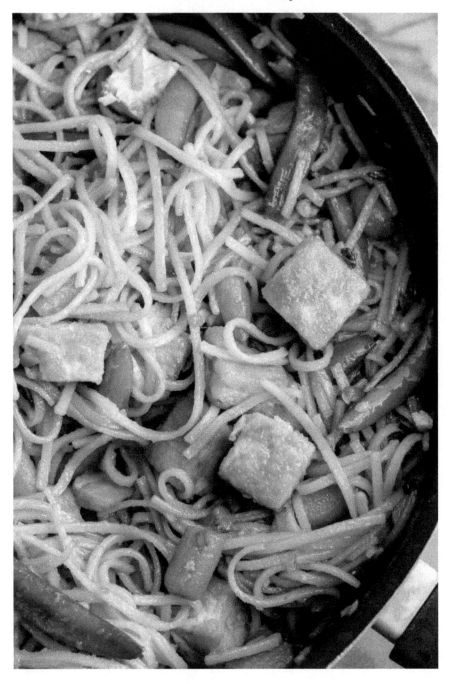

Preparation Time: 35 minutes

Serving: 4

Ingredients:

For the angel hair shirataki:

2 (8 oz) packs angel hair shirataki For the teriyaki tofu base:

2 tbsp olive oil, divided

1 ¼ lb tofu, cut into bite-size pieces Salt and black pepper to taste

1 white onion, thinly sliced

1 red bell pepper, deseeded and sliced

1 cup sliced cremini mushrooms

4 garlic cloves, minced

1 ½ cups fresh Thai basil leaves 2 tbsp toasted sesame seeds

1 tbsp chopped peanuts

1 tbsp chopped fresh scallions For the sauce:

3   tbsp coconut aminos 2 tbsp Himalayan salt

1 tbsp hot sauce

Directions:

For the angel hair shirataki:

1.   Boil 2 cups of water in a medium pot over medium heat.

2.   Strain the shirataki pasta through a colander and rinse very well under hot running water.

3.   Allow proper draining and pour the shirataki pasta into the boiling water. Cook for 3 minutes and strain again.

4.   Place a dry skillet over medium heat and stir-fry the shirataki pasta until visibly dry, and makes a squeaky sound when stirred, 1 to 2 minutes. Take off the heat and set aside.

For the teriyaki tofu base:

5.   Heat the olive oil in a large skillet, season the tofu with salt, black pepper, and sear in the oil on both sides until brown, 5 minutes. Transfer to a plate and set aside.

6.   Add the onion, bell pepper, and mushrooms to the skillet; cook until softened, 5 minutes. Stir in the garlic and cook until fragrant, 1 minute.

7.   Return the tofu to the skillet and add the pasta.

8.   Quickly, combine the sauce's Ingredients in a small bowl: coconut aminos, Himalayan salt, and hot sauce. Pour the mixture over the tofu mix. Top with the Thai basil and toss well to coat. Cook for 1 to 2 minutes or until warmed through.

9.   Dish the food onto serving plates and garnish with the sesame seeds, peanuts, and scallions.

Nutrition: Calories: 598, Total Fat: 56g, Saturated Fat:18.8g, Total Carbs: 12 g, Dietary Fiber3:g, Sugar:5 g, Protein: 15g, Sodium:762 mg

Classic Tempeh Lasagna

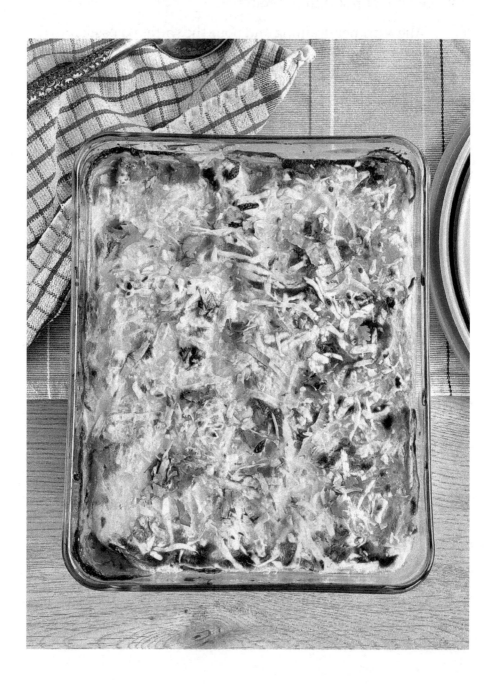

Preparation Time: 70 minutes Serving: 4

Ingredients:

For the lasagna noodles:

4   oz dairy- free cream cheese, room temperature 1 ½ cup grated mozzarella cheese

1   tsp dried Italian seasoning

2   large eggs, cracked into a bowl For the lasagna filling:

1 lb tempeh

1 medium white onion, chopped 1 tsp Italian seasoning

Salt and black pepper to taste

1 cup sugar-free marinara sauce 6 tbsp vegan ricotta cheese

½ cup grated mozzarella cheese

½ cup grated parmesan cheese

Directions:

For the lasagna noodles:

1.   Preheat the oven to 350 F and line a 9 x 13 –inch baking sheet with parchment paper.

2.   In a food processor or blender, add the dairy- free cream cheese, mozzarella cheese, Italian seasoning, and eggs. Blend until well mixed.

3.   Pour the cheese mixture on the baking sheet and spread across the pan.

4.   Bake in the middle layer of the oven until set and firm to touch, 20 minutes.

5.   Remove the cheese pasta and set aside to cool while you make the lasagna sauce. For the lasagna sauce:

6.   In a large skillet, combine the tempeh, onion and cook until brown, 5 minutes. Season with the Italian seasoning, salt, and black pepper. Cook further for 1 minute and mix in the marinara sauce. Simmer for 3 minutes. Turn the heat off.

7.   Evenly cut the lasagna pasta into thirds making sure it fits into your baking sheet.

8.   Spread a layer of the tempeh mixture in the baking sheet and make a first single layer on the tempeh mixture.

9.   Spread a third of the remaining tempeh mixture on the pasta, top with a third each of the vegan ricotta cheese, mozzarella cheese, and parmesan cheese. Repeat the layering two more times using the remaining Ingredients in the same quantities.

10.   Bake in the oven until the cheese melts and is bubbly with the sauce, 20 minutes. Serve warm

11.   Remove the lasagna, allow cooling for 2 minutes and dish onto serving plates.

Nutrition: Calories:435, Total Fat:38.3g, Saturated Fat:1.2g, Total Carbs: 4 g, Dietary Fiber:1g, Sugar: 2g,

Protein21: g, Sodium: 388mg

Creamy Sun-Dried & Parsnip Noodles

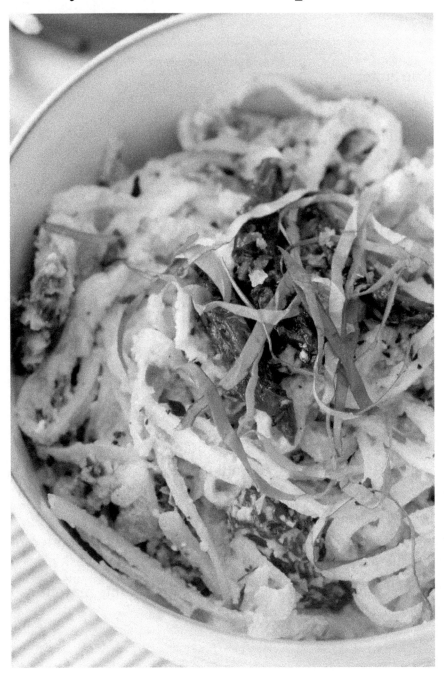

Preparation Time: 35 minutes Serving: 4

Ingredients:

3 tbsp butter

1 lb tofu, cut into strips

Salt and black pepper to taste

4 large parsnips, peeled and Blade C noodles trimmed

1 cup sun dried tomatoes in oil, chopped

4 garlic cloves, minced

1 ¼ cup coconut cream

1   cup shaved parmesan cheese

¼ tsp dried basil

¼ tsp red chili flakes

2   tbsp chopped fresh parsley for garnishing

Directions:

1.   Melt 1 tablespoon of butter in a large skillet, season the tofu with salt, black pepper and cook in the butter until brown, and cooked within, 8 to 10 minutes.

2.   In another medium skillet, melt the remaining butter and sauté the parsnips until softened, 5 to 7 minutes. Set aside.

3.   Stir in the sun-dried tomatoes and garlic into the tofu, cook until fragrant, 1 minute.

4.   Reduce the heat to low and stir in the coconut cream and parmesan cheese. Simmer until the cheese melts. Season with the salt, basil, and red chili flakes.

5.   Fold in the parsnips until well coated and cook for 2 more minutes.

6.   Dish the food into serving plates, garnish with the parsley and serve warm.

Nutrition: Calories:224, Total Fat: 20.4g, Saturated Fat:12.2 g, Total Carbs: 1 g, Dietary Fiber:0g, Sugar: 1g, Protein: 9g, Sodium:556 mg

Keto Vegan Bacon Carbonara

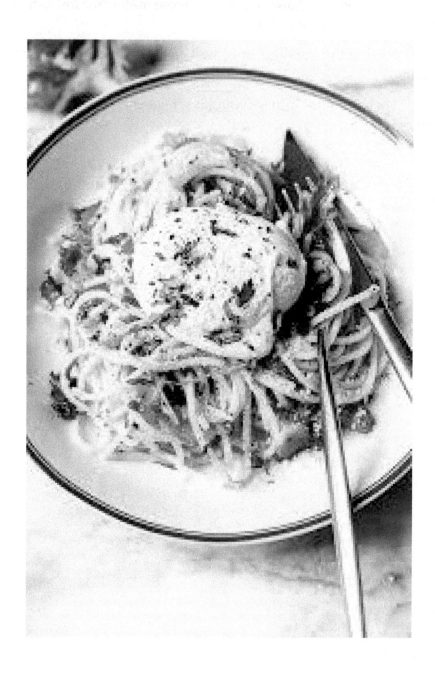

Preparation Time: 30 minutes + overnight chilling time Serving size: 4

Ingredients:

For the keto pasta:

1 cup shredded mozzarella cheese 1 large egg yolk

For the carbonara:

4 vegan bacon slices, chopped 1¼ cups coconut whipping cream

¼ cup mayonnaise

Salt and black pepper to taste 4 egg yolks

1 cup grated parmesan cheese + more for garnishing

Directions:

For the pasta:

1.   Pour the cheese into a medium safe-microwave bowl and melt in the microwave for 35 minutes or until melted.

2.   Take out the bowl and allow cooling for 1 minute only to warm the cheese but not cool completely. Mix in the egg yolk until well combined.

3.   Lay a parchment paper on a flat surface, pour the cheese mixture on top and cover with another parchment paper. Using a rolling pin, flatten the dough into 1/8-inch thickness.

4. Take off the parchment paper and cut the dough into thin spaghetti strands. Place in a bowl and refrigerate overnight.

5. When ready to cook, bring 2 cups of water to a boil in medium saucepan and add the pasta.

6. Cook for 40 seconds to 1 minute and then drain through a colander. Run cold water over the pasta and set aside to cool.

For the carbonara:

7. Add the vegan bacon to a medium skillet and cook over medium heat until crispy, 5 minutes. Set aside.

8. Pour the coconut whipping cream into a large pot and allow simmering for 3 to 5 minutes.

9. Whisk in the mayonnaise and season with the salt and black pepper. Cook for 1 minute and spoon 2 tablespoons of the mixture into a medium bowl. Allow cooling and mix in the egg yolks.

10. Pour the mixture into the pot and mix quickly until well combined. Stir in the parmesan cheese to melt and fold in the pasta.

11. Spoon the mixture into serving bowls and garnish with more parmesan cheese. Cook for 1 minute to warm the pasta.

12. Serve immediately.

Nutrition: Calories:456, Total Fat: 38.2g, Saturated Fat:14.7g, Total Carbs:13 g, Dietary Fiber:3g, Sugar: 8g, Protein:16g, Sodium:604 mg

Seitan Lo Mein

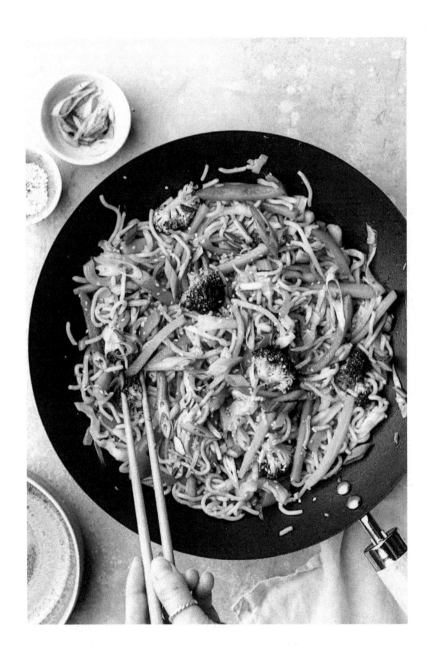

Preparation Time: 25 minutes + overtime chilling time Serving size: 4

Ingredients:

For the keto pasta:

1 cup shredded mozzarella cheese

1 egg yolk

For the seitan and vegetables:

1 tbsp sesame oil

3 seitan, cut into ¼-inch strips Salt and black pepper to taste

1 red bell pepper, deseeded and thinly sliced

1 yellow bell pepper, deseeded and thinly sliced 1 cup green beans, trimmed and halved

1 garlic clove, minced

1-inch ginger knob, peeled and grated 4 green onions, chopped

1 tsp toasted sesame seeds to garnish For the sauce:

3 tbsp coconut aminos 2 tsp sesame oil

2 tsp sugar-free maple syrup 1 tsp fresh ginger paste

Directions:

For the pasta:

1.   Pour the cheese into a medium safe-microwave bowl and melt in the microwave for 35 minutes or until melted.

2.   Take out the bowl and allow cooling for 1 minute only to warm the cheese but not cool completely. Mix in the egg yolk until well-combined.

3.   Lay a parchment paper on a flat surface, pour the cheese mixture on top and cover with another parchment paper. Using a rolling pin, flatten the dough into 1/8-inch thickness.

4.   Take off the parchment paper and cut the dough into thin spaghetti strands. Place in a bowl and refrigerate overnight.

5.   When ready to cook, bring 2 cups of water to a boil in medium saucepan and add the pasta. Cook for 40 seconds to 1 minute and then drain through a colander. Run cold water over the pasta and set aside to cool.

For the seitan and vegetables:

6.   Heat the sesame oil in a large skillet, season the seitan with salt, black pepper, and sear in the oil on both sides until brown, 5 minutes. Transfer to a plate and set aside.

7.   Mix in the bell peppers, green beans and cook until sweaty, 3 minutes. Stir in the garlic, ginger, green onions and cook until fragrant, 1 minute.

8.   Add the seitan and pasta to the skillet and toss well.

9.   In a small bowl, toss the sauce's Ingredients: the coconut aminos, sesame oil, maple syrup, and ginger paste.

10.   Pour the mixture over the seitan mixture and toss well; cook for 1 minute.

11.   Dish the food onto serving plates and garnish with the sesame seeds. Serve

warm.

Nutrition: Calories:273, Total Fat:20g, Saturated Fat:11.6g, Total Carbs:6g, Dietary Fiber:1g, Sugar:4g, Protein:17g, Sodium:931mg

Pasta & Cheese Mushroom

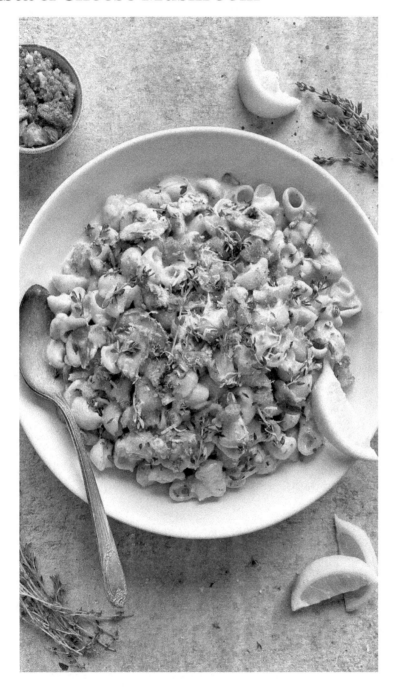

Preparation Time: 1 hour 45 minutes + overtime chilling Serving size: 4

Ingredients:

For the keto macaroni:

1 cup shredded mozzarella cheese 1 egg yolk

For the pulled mushroom mac and cheese: 2 tbsp olive oil

1 lb mushroom

Salt and black pepper to taste 1 tsp dried thyme

1   cup vegetable broth 2 tbsp butter

2   medium shallots, minced 2 garlic cloves, minced

1 cup water

1 cup grated cheddar cheese

4 oz dairy- free cream cheese, room temperature 1 cup coconut cream

½ tsp white pepper

½ tsp nutmeg powder 2 tbsp chopped parsley

Directions:

For the keto macaroni:

1.   Pour the cheese into a medium safe-microwave bowl and melt in the microwave for 35 minutes or until melted.

2.   Take out the bowl and allow cooling for 1 minute only to warm the cheese but not cool completely. Mix in the egg yolk until well-combined.

3.   Lay a parchment paper on a flat surface, pour the cheese mixture on top and cover with another parchment paper. Using a rolling pin, flatten the dough into 1/8-inch thickness.

4.   Take off the parchment paper and cut the dough into small cubes of the size of macaroni. Place in a bowl and refrigerate overnight.

5.   When ready to cook, bring 2 cups of water to a boil in medium saucepan and add the keto macaroni. Cook for 40 seconds to 1 minute and then drain through a colander. Run cold water over the pasta and set aside to cool.

For the mushroom mac and cheese:

6.   Heat the olive oil in a large pot, season the mushroom with salt, black pepper, thyme, and sear in the oil on both sides until brown. Pour on the vegetable broth, cover, and cook over low heat for 15 minutes or until softened. When ready, remove the mushroom onto a plate and set aside.

7.   Preheat the oven to 380 F.

8.   Melt the butter in a large skillet and sauté the shallots until softened. Stir in the garlic and cook until fragrant, 30 seconds.

9.   Pour in the water to deglaze the pot and then stir in half of the cheddar cheese and dairy- free cream cheese until melted, 4 minutes. Mix in the coconut cream and season with salt, black pepper, white pepper, and nutmeg powder.

10.   Add the pasta, mushroom, and half of the parsley to the mixture; combine well.

11.   Pour the mixture into a baking dish and cover the top with the remaining cheddar cheese. Bake in the oven until the cheese melts and the food bubbly, 15 to 20 minutes.

12.   Remove from the oven, allow cooling for 2 minutes and garnish with the

parsley.

13.   Serve warm.

Nutrition: Calories:647, Total Fat:56.5g, Saturated Fat:32g, Total Carbs:6g,   Dietary   Fiber:1g,   Sugar:2g,   Protein:30g, Sodium:609mg

Pesto Parmesan Tempeh with Green Pasta

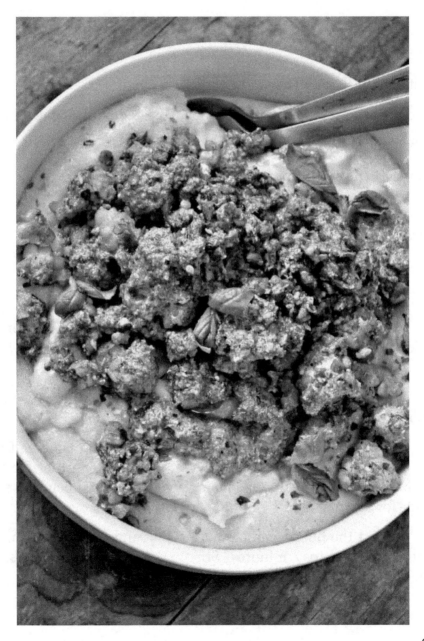

Preparation Time: 1 hour 27 minutes

Serving: 4

Ingredients:

4 tempeh

Salt and black pepper to taste

½ cup basil pesto, olive oil-based 1 cup grated parmesan cheese

1 tbsp butter

4 large turnips, Blade C, noodle trimmed

Directions:

1.   Preheat the oven to 350 F.

2.   Season the tempeh with salt, black pepper and place on a baking sheet. Divide the pesto on top and spread well on the tempeh.

3.   Place the sheet in the oven and bake for 45 minutes to 1 hour or until cooked through.

4.   When ready, pull out the baking sheet and divide half of the parmesan cheese on top of the tempeh. Cook further for 10 minutes or until the cheese melts. Remove the tempeh and set aside for serving.

5.   Melt the butter in a medium skillet and sauté the turnips until tender, 5 to 7 minutes. Stir in the remaining parmesan cheese and divide between serving plates.

6.   Top with the tempeh and serve warm.

Nutrition: Calories:442, Total Fat:29.4g, Saturated Fat:11.3g, Total Carbs:8g, Dietary Fiber:1g, Sugar:1g, Protein:39g, Sodium:814mg

Creamy Tofu with Green Beans and Keto Fettuccine

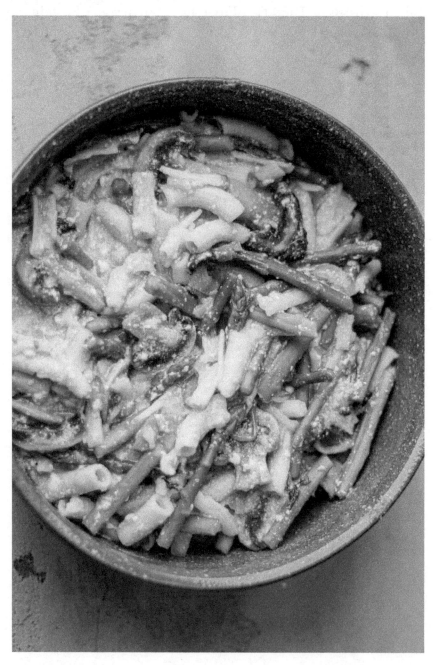

Preparation Time: 40 minutes + overtime chilling time Serving size: 4

Ingredients:

For the keto fettuccine:

1 cup shredded mozzarella cheese 1 egg yolk

For the creamy tofu and green beans:

1 tbsp olive oil

4 tofu, cut into thin strips Salt and black pepper to taste

½ cup green beans, chopped 1 lemon, zested and juiced

¼ cup vegetable broth 1 cup plain yogurt

6 basil leaves, chopped

1   cup shaved parmesan cheese for topping

Directions:

For the keto fettucine:

1.   Pour the cheese into a medium safe-microwave bowl and melt in the microwave for 35 minutes or until melted.

2.   Take out the bowl and allow cooling for 1 minute only to warm the cheese but not cool completely. Mix in the egg yolk until well-combined.

3.   Lay a parchment paper on a flat surface, pour the cheese mixture on top and cover with another parchment paper. Using a rolling pin, flatten the dough into 1/8-inch thickness.

4.   Take off the parchment paper and cut the dough into thick fettuccine strands. Place in a bowl and refrigerate overnight.

5.   When ready to cook, bring 2 cups of water to a boil in medium saucepan and add the keto fettuccine. Cook for 40 seconds to 1 minute and then drain through a colander. Run cold water over the pasta and set aside to cool.

For the creamy tofu and green beans:

6.   Heat the olive oil in a large skillet, season the tofu with salt, black pepper, and cook in the oil until brown on the outside and slightly cooked through, 10 minutes.

7.   Mix in the green beans and cook until softened, 5 minutes.

8.   Stir in the lemon zest, lemon juice, and vegetable broth. Cook for 5 more minutes or until the liquid reduces by a quarter.

9.   Add the plain yogurt and mix well. Pour in the keto fettuccine and basil, fold in well and cook for 1 minute. Adjust the taste with salt and black pepper as desired.

10.   Dish the food onto serving plates, top with the parmesan cheese and serve

warm.

Nutrition: Calories:721, Total Fat:76.8g, Saturated Fat:21.2g, Total Carbs:2g, Dietary Fiber:0g, Sugar:0g, Protein:9g, Sodium:309mg

Delicious Sambal Seitan Noodles

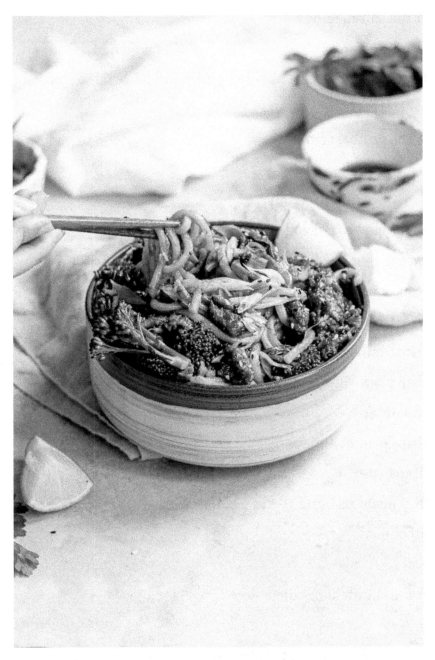

Preparation Time: 60 minutes Serving: 4

Ingredients:

For the shirataki noodles:

2 (8 oz) packs Miracle noodles, garlic and herb Salt to season

For the sambal seitan:

1 tbsp olive oil 1 lb seitan

4 garlic cloves, minced

1-inch ginger, peeled and grated 1 tsp liquid erythritol

1 tbsp sugar-free tomato paste

2   fresh basil leaves + extra for garnishing

2 tbsp sambal oelek

2 tbsp plain vinegar

1 cup water

2 tbsp coconut aminos

Salt to taste

1 tbsp unsalted butter

 Directions:

For the shirataki noodles:

1.   Bring 2 cups of water to a boil in a medium pot over medium heat.

2.   Strain the Miracle noodles through a colander and rinse very well under hot running water.

3.   Allow proper draining and pour the noodles into the boiling water. Cook for 3 minutes and strain again.

4.   Place a dry skillet over medium heat and stir-fry the shirataki noodles until visibly dry, 1 to 2 minutes. Season with salt, plate and set aside.

For the seitan sambal:

5.   Heat the olive oil in a large pot and cook in the seitan until brown, 5 minutes.

6.   Stir in the garlic, ginger, liquid erythritol and cook for 1 minute.

7.   Add the tomato paste, cook for 2 minutes and mix in the basil, sambal oelek, vinegar, water, coconut aminos, and salt. Cover the pot and continue cooking over low heat for 30 minutes.

8.   Uncover, add the shirataki noodles, butter and mix well into the sauce.

9.   Dish the food, garnish with some basil leaves and serve warm.

Nutrition: Calories:538, Total Fat:41.1g, Saturated Fat:16.2g, Total Carbs:20g, Dietary Fiber:14g, Sugar:5g, Protein:29g, Sodium:640mg

Tofu Avocado Keto Noodles

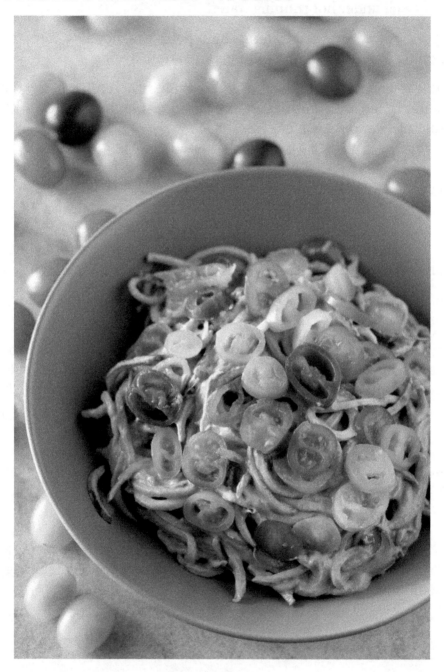

Preparation Time: 15 minutes Serving: 4

Ingredients:

2 tbsp butter

1 lb tofu

Salt and black pepper to taste

8 large red and yellow bell peppers, Blade A, noodles trimmed 1 tsp garlic powder

2 medium avocados, pitted, peeled and mashed 2 tbsp chopped pecans for topping

Directions:

1.   Melt the butter in a large skillet and cook the tofu until brown, 5 minutes. Season with salt and black pepper.

2.   Stir in the bell peppers, garlic powder and cook until the peppers are slightly tender, 2 minutes.

3.   Mix in the mashed avocados, adjust the taste with salt and black pepper and cook for 1 minute.

4.   Dish the food onto serving plates, garnish with the pecans and serve warm.

Nutrition: Calories:209, Total Fat:15.2g, Saturated Fat:7.3g, Total Carbs:8g, Dietary Fiber:1g, Sugar:2g, Protein:13g, Sodium:468mg

Lemongrass Tempeh with Spaghetti Squash

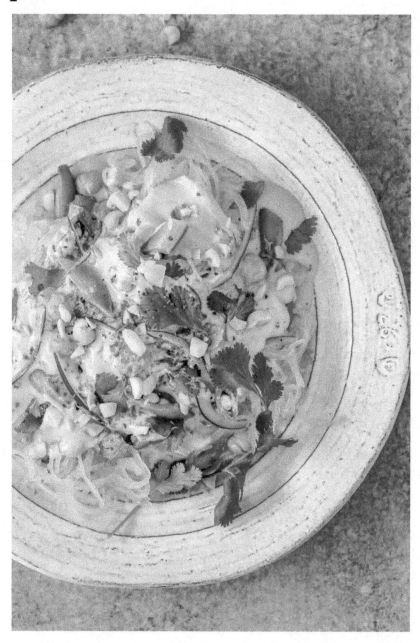

Preparation Time: 1 hour + 45 minutes marinating time Serving size: 4

Ingredients:

For the lemongrass tempeh:

2 tbsp minced lemongrass 2 tbsp fresh ginger paste

2 tbsp sugar-free maple syrup 2 tbsp coconut aminos

1   tbsp Himalayan salt 4 tempeh

2   tbsp avocado oil For the squash noodles:

3   lb spaghetti squashes, halved and deseeded 1 tbsp olive oil

Salt and black pepper to taste For the steamed spinach:

1 tbsp avocado oil

1 tsp fresh ginger paste 1 lb baby spinach

For the peanut-coconut sauce:

½ cup coconut milk

¼ cup organic almond butter

Directions:

For the lemongrass tempeh:

1.   In a medium bowl, mix the lemongrass, ginger paste, maple syrup, coconut aminos, and Himalayan salt. Place the tempeh in the liquid and coat well. Allow marinating for 45 minutes.

2.   After, heat the avocado oil in a large skillet, remove the tempeh from the marinade and sear in the oil on both sides until golden brown and cooked through, 10 to 15 minutes. Transfer to a plate and cover with foil.

For the spaghetti squash:

3.   Preheat the oven to 380 F.

4.   Place the spaghetti squashes on a baking sheet, brush with the olive oil and season with salt and black pepper. Bake in the oven for 20 to 25 minutes or until tender.

5.   When ready, remove the squash and shred with two forks into spaghetti-like strands. Keep warm in the oven.

For the spinach:

6.   In another skillet, heat the avocado oil and sauté the ginger until fragrant. Add the spinach and cook to wilt while stirring to be coated well in the ginger, 2 minutes. Turn the heat off.

For the almond-coconut sauce:

7.   In a medium bowl, quickly whisk the coconut milk with the almond butter until well combined.

8.   To serve:

9.   Unwrap and divide the tempeh into four bowls, add the spaghetti squash to the side, then the spinach and drizzle the almond sauce on top.

10.   Serve immediately.

Nutrition: Calories:457, Total Fat:37g, Saturated Fat:8.1g, Total Carbs:17g, Dietary Fiber:5g, Sugar:4g,

Protein:22g, Sodium:656mg

Pear and Arugula Salad

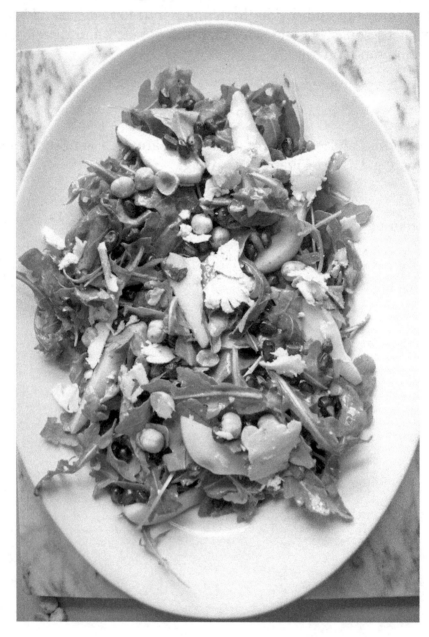

Preparation Time: 10 Minutes Cooking Time: 8 Minutes
Servings:4

Ingredients

¼ cup chopped pecans 10 ounces arugula

2   pears, thinly sliced

1 tablespoon finely minced shallot

2 tablespoons champagne vinegar

2 tablespoons olive oil

¼ teaspoon sea salt

¼ teaspoon freshly ground black pepper

¼ teaspoon dijon mustard

Directions

1.   Preheat the oven to 350°F.

2.   Spread the pecans in a single layer on a baking sheet. Toast in the preheated oven until fragrant, about 6 minutes. Remove from the oven and let cool. In a large bowl, toss the pecans, arugula, and pears. In a small bowl, whisk together the shallot, vinegar, olive oil, salt, pepper, and mustard. Toss with the salad and serve immediately.

Quinoa Salad With Black Beans And Tomatoes

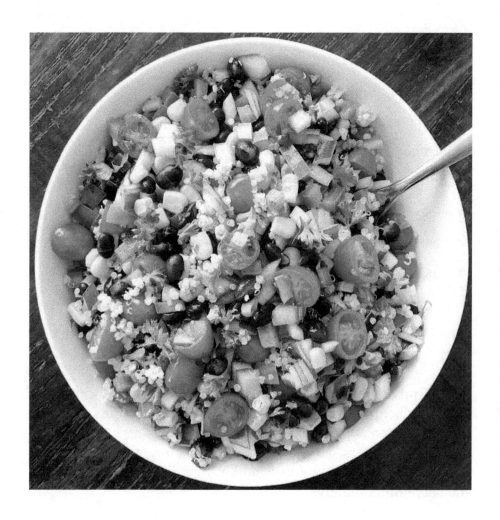

Preparation Time: 5 Minutes Cooking Time: 20 Minutes Servings:4

Ingredients

3 cups water

1½ cups quinoa, well rinsed

Salt

1½ cups cooked or 1 (15.5-ounce) can black beans, drained and rinsed 4 ripe plum tomatoes, cut into ¼-inch dice

⅓ cup minced red onion

¼ cup chopped fresh parsley

¼ cup olive oil

2 tablespoons sherry vinegar

¼ teaspoon freshly ground black pepper

Directions

1.   In a large saucepan, bring the water to boil over high heat. Add the quinoa, salt the water, and return to a boil. Reduce heat to low, cover, and simmer until the water is absorbed, about 20 minutes.

2.   Transfer the cooked quinoa to a large bowl. Add the black beans, tomatoes, onion, and parsley.

3.   In a small bowl, combine the olive oil, vinegar, salt to taste, and pepper. Pour the dressing over the salad and toss well to combine. Cover and set aside for 20 minutes before serving.

Mediterranean Quinoa Salad

Preparation Time: 5 Minutes Cooking Time: 20 Minutes Servings:4

Ingredients

2 cups water

1   cup quinoa, well rinsed Salt

1½ cups cooked or 1 (15.5-ounce) can chickpeas, drained and rinsed 1 cup ripe grape or cherry tomatoes, halved

2   green onions, minced

½ medium English cucumber, peeled and chopped

¼ cup pitted brine-cured black olives

2 tablespoons toasted pine nuts ¼ cup small fresh basil leaves 1 medium shallot, chopped

1 garlic clove, chopped

1   teaspoon Dijon mustard

2   tablespoons white wine vinegar

¼ cup olive oil

Freshly ground black pepper

Directions

1.   In a large saucepan, bring the water to boil over high heat. Add the quinoa, salt the water, and return to a boil. Reduce heat to low, cover, and simmer until water is absorbed, about 20 minutes.

2.　Transfer the cooked quinoa to a large bowl. Add the chickpeas, tomatoes, green onions, cucumber, olives, pine nuts, and basil. Set aside.

3.　In a blender or food processor, combine the shallot, garlic, mustard, vinegar, oil, and salt and pepper to taste. Process until well blended. Pour the dressing over the salad, toss gently to combine, and serve.

Apple, Pecan, and Arugula Salad

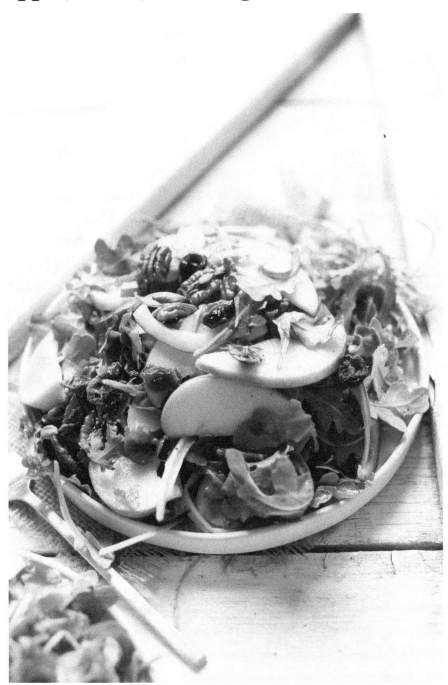

Preparation Time: 10 Minutes Cooking Time: 0 Minutes
Servings:4

Ingredients

Juice of 1 lemon

2 tablespoons olive oil

1 tablespoon maple syrup

2 pinches sea salt

1 (5-ounce) package arugula

1   cup frozen (and thawed) or fresh corn kernels

½ red onion, thinly sliced

2   apples (preferably Gala or Fuji), cored and sliced

½ cup chopped pecans

¼ cup dried cranberries

Directions

1.   In a small bowl, whisk together the lemon juice, oil, maple syrup, and salt. In a large bowl, combine the arugula, corn, red onion, and apples. Add the lemon-juice mixture and toss to combine.

2.   Divide evenly among 4 plates and top with the pecans and cranberries.

Caesar Salad

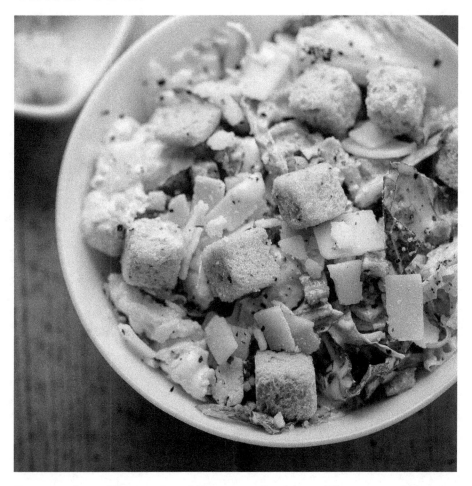

Preparation Time: 10 Minutes Cooking Time: 0 Minutes
Servings:1

Ingredients

For The Caesar Salad

2 cups chopped romaine lettuce

2 tablespoons

Caesar Dressing

1 serving Herbed Croutons or store-bought croutons

Vegan cheese, grated (optional)

Make It A Meal

½ cup cooked pasta

½ cup canned chickpeas, drained and rinsed 2 additional tablespoons Caesar Dressing

Directions

1.   To Make The Caesar Salad. In a large bowl, toss together the lettuce, dressing, croutons, and cheese (if using).

2.   To Make It A Meal. Add the pasta, chickpeas, and additional dressing. Toss to coat.

Per Serving (in a meal) Calories: 415; Protein: 19g; Total fat: 8g; Saturated fat: 1g; Carbohydrates: 72g; Fiber: 13g

Classic Potato Salad

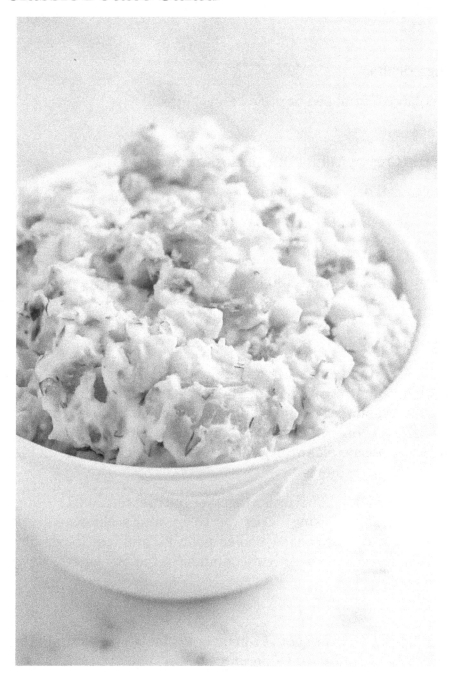

Preparation Time: 10 Minutes Cooking Time: 15 Minutes Servings:4

Ingredients

6 potatoes, scrubbed or peeled and chopped

Pinch salt

½ cup Creamy Tahini Dressing or vegan mayo

1 teaspoon dried dill (optional)

1   teaspoon Dijon mustard (optional)

4 celery stalks, chopped

2   scallions, white and light green parts only, chopped

Directions

1.   Put the potatoes in a large pot, add the salt, and pour in enough water to cover. Bring the water to a boil over high heat. Cook the potatoes for 15 to 20 minutes, until soft. Drain and set aside to cool. (Alternatively, put the potatoes in a large microwave-safe dish with a bit of water. Cover and heat on high power for 10 minutes.)

2.   In a large bowl, whisk together the dressing, dill (if using), and mustard (if using). Toss the celery and scallions with the dressing. Add the cooked, cooled potatoes and toss to combine. Store leftovers in an airtight container in the refrigerator for up to 1 week.

Per Serving Calories: 269; Protein: 6g; Total fat: 5g; Saturated fat: 1g; Carbohydrates: 51g; Fiber: 6g

Brown Rice and Pepper Salad

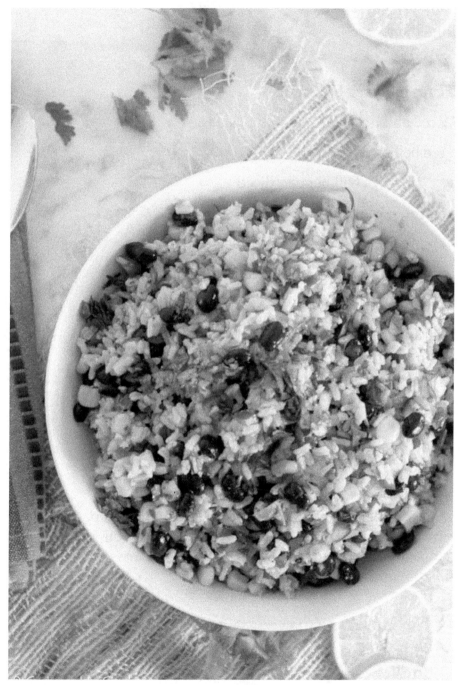

Preparation Time: 15 Minutes Cooking Time: 0 Minutes Servings:4

Ingredients

2 cups prepared brown rice

½ red onion, diced

1 red bell pepper, diced

1   orange bell pepper, diced

1 carrot, diced

¼ cup olive oil

2   tablespoons unseasoned rice vinegar

1 tablespoon soy sauce

1 garlic clove, minced

1   tablespoon grated fresh ginger

¼ teaspoon sea salt

¼ teaspoon freshly ground black pepper

Directions

1.   In a large bowl, combine the rice, onion, bell peppers, and carrot. In a small bowl, whisk together the olive oil, rice vinegar, soy sauce, garlic, ginger, salt, and pepper. Toss with the rice mixture and serve immediately.

Mediterranean Orzo & Chickpea Salad

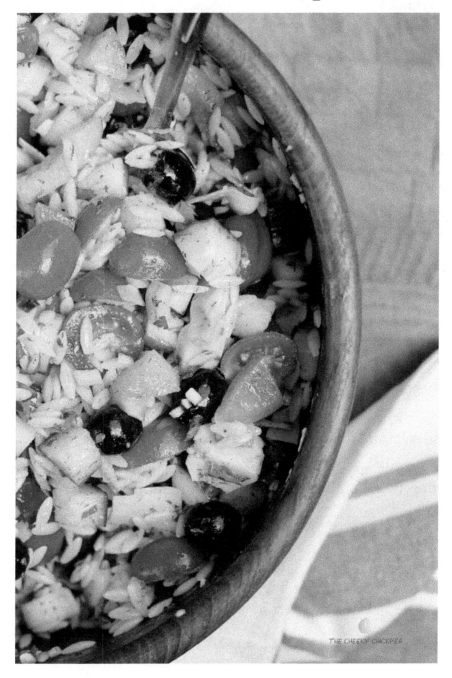

Preparation Time: 15 Minutes Cooking Time: 8 Minutes
Servings:4

Ingredients

¼ cup olive oil

2   tablespoons freshly squeezed lemon juice

Pinch salt

1½ cups canned chickpeas, drained and rinsed

2 cups orzo or other small pasta shape, cooked according to the
package directions, drained, and rinsed with cold water to cool

2 cups raw spinach, finely chopped

1 cup chopped cucumber

¼ red onion, finely diced

Directions

1.   In a large bowl, whisk together the olive oil, lemon juice,
and salt. Add the chickpeas and cooked orzo, and toss to coat.

2.   Stir in the spinach, cucumber, and red onion. Store
leftovers in an airtight container in the refrigerator for up to 5
days.

Per Serving Calories: 233; Protein: 6g; Total fat: 15g; Saturated
fat: 2g; Carbohydrates: 20g; Fiber: 5g

Roasted Carrot Salad

Preparation Time: 10 Minutes Cooking Time: 30 Minutes Servings:3

Ingredients

4 carrots, peeled and sliced

1 to 2 teaspoons olive oil or coconut oil

½ teaspoon ground cinnamon or pumpkin pie spice Salt

1 (15-ounce) can cannellini beans or navy beans, drained and rinsed

3 cups chopped hearty greens, such as spinach, kale, chard, or collards

⅓ cup dried cranberries or pomegranate seeds

⅓ cup slivered almonds or Cinnamon-Lime Sunflower Seeds

¼ cup Raspberry Vinaigrette or Cilantro-Lime Dressing, or 2 tablespoons freshly squeezed orange or lemon juice whisked with 2 tablespoons olive oil and a pinch of salt

Directions

1.

Preheat the oven or toaster oven to 400°F.

2.   In a medium bowl, toss the carrots with the olive oil and cinnamon and season to taste with salt. Transfer to a small tray, and roast for 15 minutes or until browned around the edges. Toss the carrots, add the beans, and roast for 15 minutes more. Let cool while you prep the salad. Divide the greens among three plates or

containers, top with the cranberries and almonds, and add the roasted carrots and beans.

3.   Drizzle with the dressing of your choice. Store leftovers in an airtight container in the refrigerator for up to 1 week.

Roasted Potato Salad With Chickpeas And Tomatoes

Preparation Time: 5 Minutes Cooking Time: 20 Minutes Servings:4 To 6

Ingredients

1½ pounds Yukon Gold potatoes, cut into ½-inch dice

1 medium shallot, halved lengthwise and cut into ¼-inch slices ¼ cup olive oil

Salt and freshly ground black pepper 3 tablespoons white wine vinegar

1½ cups cooked or 1 (15.5-ounce) can chickpeas, drained and rinsed ⅓ cup chopped drained oil-packed sun-dried tomatoes

¼ cup green olives, pitted and halved ¼ cup chopped fresh parsley

Directions

1.   Preheat the oven to 425°F. In a large bowl, combine the potatoes, shallot, and 1 tablespoon of the oil. Season with salt and pepper to taste and toss to coat. Transfer the potatoes and shallot to a baking sheet and roast, turning once, until tender and golden brown, about 20 minutes. Transfer to a large bowl and set aside to cool.

2.   In a small bowl, combine the remaining 3 tablespoons oil with the vinegar and pepper to taste. Add the chickpeas, tomatoes, olives, and parsley to the cooked potatoes and shallots. Drizzle with the dressing and toss gently to combine. Taste, adjusting seasonings if necessary. Serve warm or at room temperature.

Spinach and Pomegranate Salad

Preparation Time: 10 Minutes Cooking Time: 0 Minutes
Servings:4

Ingredients

10 ounces baby spinach seeds from 1 pomegranate

1 cup fresh blackberries

¼ red onion, thinly sliced

½ cup chopped pecans

¼ cup balsamic vinegar

¾ cup olive oil

½ teaspoon sea salt

½ teaspoon freshly ground black pepper

Directions

1.   In a large bowl, combine the spinach, pomegranate seeds, blackberries, red onion, and pecans.

2.   In a small bowl, whisk together the vinegar, olive oil, salt, and pepper. Toss with the salad and serve immediately.

Cobb Salad with Portobello Bacon

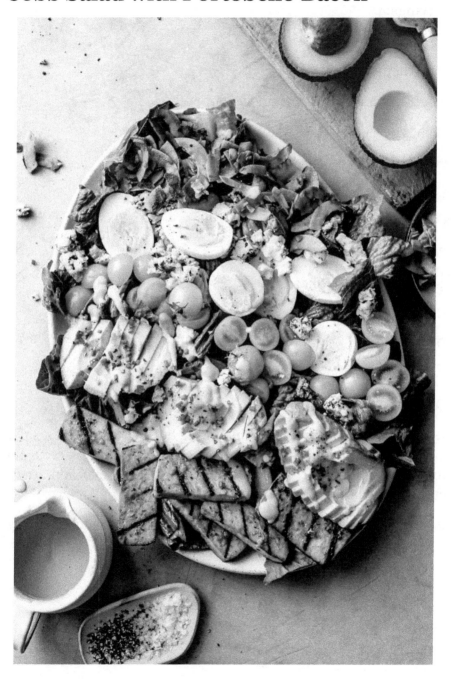

Preparation Time: 15 Minutes Cooking Time: 0 Minutes Servings:4

Ingredients

2 heads romaine lettuce, finely chopped

1 pint cherry tomatoes, halved

1 avocado, peeled, pitted, and diced

1 cup frozen (and thawed) or fresh corn kernels

1 large cucumber, peeled and diced

Portobello Bacon or store-bought vegan bacon

4 scallions, thinly sliced

Unhidden Valley Ranch

Dressing or store-bought vegan ranch dressing

Directions

1.   Scatter a layer of romaine in the bottom of each of 4 salad bowls. With the following ingredients, create lines that cross the top of the romaine, in this order: tomatoes, avocado, corn, cucumber, and portobello bacon.

2.   Sprinkle with the scallions and drizzle with ranch dressing.

German-Style Potato Salad

Preparation Time: 15 Minutes Cooking Time: 0 Minutes Servings:4 To 6

Ingredients

1½ pounds white potatoes, unpeeled

½ cup olive oil

4 slices tempeh bacon, homemade or store-bought

1 medium bunch green onions, chopped

1 tablespoon whole-wheat flour

2 tablespoons sugar

⅓ cup white wine vinegar

¼ cup water

½ teaspoon salt

⅛ teaspoon freshly ground black pepper

Directions

1.　In a large pot of boiling salted water, cook the potatoes until just tender, about 30 minutes. Drain well and set aside to cool.

2.　In a large skillet, heat the oil over medium heat. Add the tempeh bacon and cook until browned on both sides, about 5 minutes total. Remove from skillet, and set aside to cool.

3.　Cut the cooled potatoes into 1-inch chunks and place in a large bowl. Crumble or chop the cooked tempeh bacon and add to the potatoes.

4. Reheat the skillet over medium heat. Add the green onions and cook for 1 minute to soften. Stir in the flour, sugar, vinegar, water, salt, and pepper, and bring to a boil, stirring until smooth. Pour the hot dressing onto the potatoes. Stir gently to combine and serve.

Sweet Pearl Couscous Salad with Pear & Cranberries

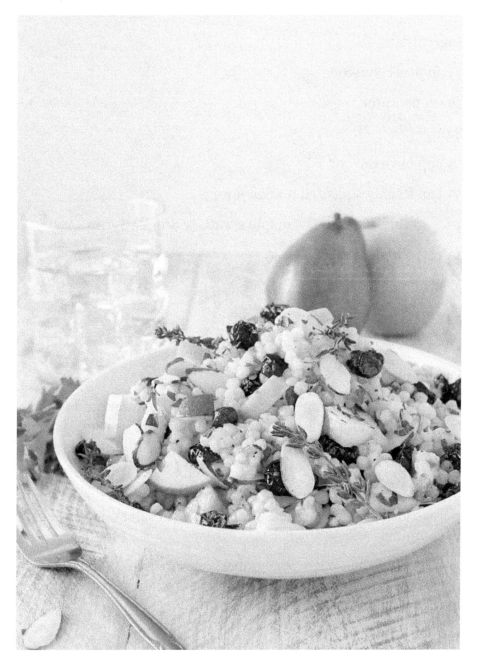

Preparation Time: 5 Minutes Cooking Time: 10 Minutes
Servings:4

Ingredients

1 cup pearl couscous

1½ cups water

Salt

¼ cup olive oil

¼ cup freshly squeezed orange juice

1   tablespoon sugar, maple syrup, or Simple Syrup

1 pear, cored and diced

½ cucumber, diced

¼ cup dried cranberries or raisins

Directions

1.   In a small pot, combine the couscous, water, and a pinch of salt. Bring to a boil over high heat, turn the heat to low, and cover the pot. Simmer for about 10 minutes, until the couscous is al dente.

2.   Meanwhile, in a large bowl, whisk together the olive oil, orange juice, and sugar. Season to taste with salt and whisk again to combine.

3.   Add the pear, cucumber, cranberries, and cooked couscous. Toss to combine. Store leftovers in an airtight container in the refrigerator for up to 1 week.

Per Serving Calories: 365; Protein: 6g; Total fat: 14g; Saturated fat: 2g; Carbohydrates: 55g; Fiber: 4g

Lightning Source UK Ltd.
Milton Keynes UK
UKHW022032060521
383282UK00003B/319